The 5:2 Vegetarian Diet Made eZy

Polly Fielding

Copyright © 2013 Polly Fielding

www.pollyfielding.com

ISBN-13: 978-1491065907

ISBN-10: 1491065907

Also by Polly Fielding

And This Is My Adopted Daughter
*The powerful true story of an adopted child's relationship with
 two mothers*

A Mind To Be Free
 The minefield of the mental health system

Crossing The Borderline
Inside a therapeutic community

Letting Go
 A trilogy comprising the three books listed above

The 5:2 Diet Made eZy

Going In Seine
An apartment in Paris? You must be joking!

Missing Factor
A personal experience of haemophilia

To Simon, Rachel, Nathan, Benjamin and Joel
who have brought such joy into my life

CONTENTS

The picture on the cover of this book was created by the author. It is not a serving suggestion!

What is the 5:2 Diet?

The 5:2 way of eating is an easily-understood concept. You simply choose any two days per week – alternated, consecutive or a few days apart – and for each of those two days, whatever you put into your mouth should amount to a total 500 calories for a woman or 600 for a man. On the other five days you eat and drink whatever you normally would. Restricted calorie days are often referred to as "fast" days and the other five are called "feed" days. This diet is also known as the Intermittent Fasting Diet or Fast Diet. It is *fast* in the sense that the positive results of this increasingly popular style of eating show up pretty quickly!

Although the number of calories consumed on the two "fast" days is restricted it is entirely up to you how you divide it up. So, for example, someone might choose to have a breakfast of 200 calories, nothing for lunch and 300/400 calories (depending on your gender) for dinner; whilst another might skip breakfast and spread the allocation over the other two meals; or yet again, you may prefer very light snacks at regular intervals throughout the day.

Whichever way you do it you may be concerned about over-eating on the "feed" days to compensate. However, those who are on this diet rarely find this to be the case.

Scientific data so far seems to indicate a number of significant health benefits to using the 5:2 method. Not only does it suggest that it can result in steady weight loss, but apparently it can also improve blood sugar levels and reduce cholesterol. Moreover, the risk of serious illnesses such as heart disease, cancer and diabetes can be considerably lessened. In addition, some scientists claim that following the 5:2 diet can protect the brain against diseases like Alzheimer's and Parkinson's and improve cognitive function, keeping us mentally more alert for longer. It is believed that controlling the level of a hormone known as IGF-1 through fasting can even lead to extended longevity. IGF-1 is important in youth for growth but as we get older high levels appear to work against us, hastening the aging process and increasing susceptibility to age-related diseases.

The main evidence for this comes from the intensive research into a condition known as Laron Syndrome (named after the Israeli researcher who first identified it). Those born with this rare disorder – 250 reported cases worldwide – are deficient in the insulin-related growth hormone which means that they do not reach above three and a half feet in height as fully grown adults. However, the upside of this condition is that, not only do they not develop serious conditions such as diabetes, cancer or brain deterioration that the rest of the human race is susceptible to, but (barring fatal accidents) they all live to a ripe old age.

The good news for anyone on the 5:2 diet is that fasting lowers the amount of this hormone and puts the body into "repair mode" by slowing down the production of new cells and repairing existing ones instead. So it is possible to undo some of the damage we may have done to ourselves. And who doesn't want to look younger and be healthier for longer?

Studies on aging reveal that fasting once or twice a week does indeed lower IGF-1 levels, which encourages fat-burning. And there are some very long-living, active, alert and healthy mice to prove it.

However, critics of the 5:2 diet say there have been insufficient studies with human beings to categorically state its long-term positive or potential harmful effects. Some nutritionists have expressed concern about the diet possibly triggering eating disorders, though it could be argued that this could be well be the case with any diet taken to extremes.

Traditionally, there has been a lot of emphasis on the need for exercise to keep us healthy; but whilst some exercise is good for us to improve our over-all health and muscle tone, there are medics who believe that too much can eventually be detrimental to health. The ideal recipe would seem to be a combination of moderate exercise and a well-thought-out diet.

All advocates of the 5:2 diet agree that plenty of water intake is essential to avoid digestive and constipation problems. Water also lessens hunger, rehydrates the body and improves the skin. Surprisingly, it has even been proposed that drinking water is quite possibly the single, most important catalyst in losing weight and keeping it off. So no harm in drinking eight glasses a day then! And it's all calorie-free!

Why and How I Started

I first heard about the 5:2 diet whilst watching an episode of Horizon, a UK science documentary television series. This particular programme was about dieting, a subject that particularly interests me.

Munching on a packet of crisps washed down with a couple of glasses of wine, I was rapidly losing interest. The sight of a tired and strained Doctor Michael Mosley, the programme's presenter, sitting on a sunny Los Angeles beach whilst following a three-day, four-night fast, spoiled my enjoyment of my snack. He was not allowed to ingest anything other than lots of water, black tea and one 50 calorie cup-a-soup per day.

This was not a one-off fast; it would need to be repeated every couple of months to retain the beneficial results that a battery of health tests had revealed when he finished his fast.

I was just about to switch off when Dr Mosley announced rather downheartedly that using this method to lose weight and become healthier was not a life-long option he was prepared to undertake. He was determined to see whether any other, hopefully less stringent, route could maintain the same healthier results he'd achieved with his drastic fast.

He did indeed find a more palatable way that did not

involve resorting to prolonged fasting. At the Institute for Aging in Baltimore, Maryland, he was taken to see some mice that had been reared on "feast" and "fast" days – or "intermittent energy restriction days" as they were also termed. They were living much longer, showed far less risk of the early onset of brain disease than the control group and demonstrated far better memory recall in tests.

The researchers concluded that hunger really does make the brain sharper; and when questioned about the possibility of comparable results in humans following a similar regime, they said that the chances are very good to excellent of slowing down the aging process and giving many more years of healthy living.

In the interests of science and his own wellbeing, Dr Mosley practised the 5:2 diet over a five-week period.

The positive improvements were dramatic. Tests showed that his blood-sugar and cholesterol levels were now normal, whereas before he was bordering diabetic and might soon have to start medication to control his cholesterol level. And his IGF-1 had reduced by fifty percent, greatly lowering his risk of cancers and diminishing the risk of dementia. These were life-changing results and Dr Mosley expressed his intention to continue eating this way.

I was sufficiently impressed that by the end of the programme I had already formed my intention to begin the 5:2 diet. Whatever diet I've previously tried has lasted at most a week before I've reverted to attempts to generally eat better, sticking to healthier cooking oils and bread spreads and eating lots of fruit and vegetables. But still, those stubborn extra pounds I had accumulated over the years refused to drop off – and worse, I felt guilty every time I ate a bar of chocolate, a cream cake or even the biscuit crumbs at the bottom of the tin.

The idea of restricting my calorie intake on just a couple of days a week, in fact any two days of my choice, and having more or less what I fancied on the other five, had, and still has, immense appeal.

I must admit, I was rather sceptical about eating *anything* I wanted on my unrestricted-calorie days. So, although allowing myself ice-cream, baguettes and chocolate biscuits, I resolved to avoid the usual guilty feelings when consuming my favourite foods by including a good balance of fruit and vegetables and going for a brisk walk or visiting the gym more often.

The day after making my decision, wasting no time I plunged into a "fast" day. I ate no breakfast, had an apple for lunch and so saved most of my calories for my evening meal. With a raging headache, due to insufficient water intake, and gnawing hunger pains, I spent most of the evening trying to figure out the correct number of calories per hundred grams for foods I had in stock, desperate to make a nutritious meal. By 9.30pm, when I had finally cobbled together a mixed salad with some cheese, I was utterly exhausted and confused about how many calories I had actually consumed that day.

Hours spent researching calorific values on various websites of a particular food item showed quite wide variations. And how was I even supposed to know how the authors arrived at the total number of calories for an omelette, for example, when the calories for individual ingredients were not specified.

My disorganised approach continued for the next couple of "fast" days. On day two, having eaten what I thought was a small breakfast, a medium-sized lunch and drunk a few cups of tea with semi-skimmed milk, I totted up the calories and found that I'd used up my allotted 500 and had none left for the rest of the day. My husband did not fail to notice how bad-tempered I became while starving my body for the remainder of that day.

On the third day I got to the point where I had one calorie left for the day, which, in my intense desire to be mathematically accurate in my calorie consumption for the day, I was determined to use up. So I decided to eat one very small inner leaf of a Cos lettuce. I kidded myself that its laudanum content would help me sleep better. Later, however, I had a reality check and realised that it would actually take at least a kilo of lettuce to make a significant impact!

Day four was equally, though differently, disastrous.

I won't bore you with the details. Suffice it to say that I grossly exceeded my intended calorie intake.

I finally took stock, scheduled Monday and Thursday for my two "fast" days the following week and set about planning a structured, commonsense approach, one that would make life easy and not involve panicking or obsessing on my two low-calorie days. And instead of weighing myself on a daily basis I decided to limit myself to once a week. I resolved to integrate enjoyment and fun into the journey to becoming a healthier me.

I also realised that I would need to target my plan to match the goals of the mnemonic SMART – i.e. it would have to be:

Specific

Measurable

Attainable

Relevant

Time-limited

This last goal triggered in me a sense of urgency, excitement and revived my waning enthusiasm.

About This Book

After what was clearly a very confusing start to my attempt to embrace the 5:2 diet, which almost culminated in me consigning it to history, along with the other diets I've tried, I sat down and worked out a different approach: a **SMART** plan. I realised I needed to feel at ease with the whole process. To that end I would stop regarding the 5:2 diet as "fasting" and "feeding" days. Fasting sounds to me somewhat punitive, a form of self-deprivation – and I'm not masochistic. So in future these would be known as LoCal days; I'm comfortable with that and it's a more accurate description. Meanwhile, "feeding" does not convey the pleasure of relaxed eating and drinking. So I prefer to regard those five days as "Indulgence" days. This does not mean doing everything to excess but simply making eating and drinking enjoyable experiences.

I no longer wanted to devote a large chunk of each day to working out afresh the calorific content of everything I ate or drank. I decided instead to invest time in devising a counter, which would ultimately simplify the entire process; it can be found at the end of this book, together with an alphabetical chart. The groundwork would then be done as far as calorie-counting was concerned and I could mix and match according to my tastes and calorie requirements.

One area of confusion occurred when I tried to find out why the packaging on many foods refers to calories as "kcal". The k is short for kilo, which means a thousand. A thousand calories? Does this mean that my innocent 20 calorie Ryvita crispbread slice actually contains 20,000 calories? Surely not! I looked the whole thing up on Wikipedia and discovered the scientific facts, which made my eyes glaze over a bit. All I need to report here is that for all practical, weight-watching purposes, "kcal" and "cal" mean the same thing as far as we are concerned, even if to a scientist they are different. So if you read on a packet that a meal contains 300kcal, that's 300 calories to you and me.

I am no gourmet chef. I don't dine on such "delicacies" as truffles, whatever their calorific value – and anyway, I doubt whether my local supermarket would stock them. Besides, I'm not prepared to spend time and money collecting either expensive or rare ingredients to make a meal, especially as I don't even know whether I'd like them. Moreover, if I were to be suddenly seized by an overwhelming desire to try these on my Indulgence days, I could always visit an upmarket restaurant.

Over the course of twelve weeks, I did my research on grams and calories and devised meals for the twenty-four LoCal days in that period with as much variation of diet as possible and as little preparation as I could get away with. This also avoided the need to linger in the kitchen with the possible temptation of helping myself to "snacks" from the cupboards! The keynote had to be Simplicity as I got to grips with the 5:2 diet. I reckoned that after twelve weeks I could begin the cycle again.

This method would avoid the boredom factor which is often a turn-off in any diet plan. A friend of mine commented that she always had a 50 calorie cup soup for lunch and a ready-prepared calorie-counted meal from the supermarket on her LoCal days; but she soon ran out of choice and constant shopping for the correct calorie ready meals swallowed up too much time of her busy day as well as proving rather costly.

I showed her the notes I had made so far for myself and she said, "That's just what I need! Can I have a copy?" At that point I realised I had the basis of a book. A book for other people like me, who want to follow a diet but who also want a life.

And this is it.

How you organise your LoCal days should be your choice. However, my mood became affected when I left almost all my calorie intake until the evening and my blood sugar dropped owing to hunger, leaving me feeling quite faint and shaky. So I have tried to spread food intake somewhat more evenly over the day. Plus I tend to have my evening meal reasonably early and avoid getting to bed late. The result is a far less hungry and happier me. I would suggest you take a similar approach.

I also find that a glass of water, especially just before a meal, often relieves the urge to eat too much as it dampens down my hunger response. I drink on average a litre and a half per day throughout the week, even on Indulgence days.

I initially thought that after a LoCal day I would inevitably consume ten times the usual amount of food on my non-restricted days. My personal experience has shown this not to be the case. Before beginning the 5:2 diet, I wasn't really considering whether I actually wanted and/or appreciated everything I consumed in a day. It was only when I paid attention to what I ate and drank that my body had a chance to let me know that I'd had enough. Previously, I just used to plough on without listening to my body, stuffing in anything and everything, so to speak.

Another enormous plus of my new way of life was that I became increasingly aware of the taste of each morsel of food. I also began to savour the smell, texture and colour of everything I ingested. This makes the experience of eating and drinking so much more pleasurable. Additionally, I now eat considerably more slowly, which gives me the opportunity to notice flavours, appearance, presentation.... as well as being the more favourable way for my body to digest food. The next chapter explores this in more detail.

At the start of each week I plan my two LoCal days,

spacing them out to suit myself so that, for example, if I have a wedding to attend or I am going out to a restaurant, that day will not be one of them.

I am consciously enjoying my meals, no longer eating out of boredom or habit; and, with little effort, I have shifted ten pounds (4½ kilos) in twelve weeks, bringing my weight so far down to a reasonably healthy level for my age and height, without taking drastic measures.

I have found that it is best to have my once-weekly weigh-in first thing in the morning before getting dressed. And if, occasionally, I gain slightly more weight (like when I went on holiday and had a week of no low calorie days) I don't stress about it as I know the pounds will drop off again as soon I return to keeping to my two LoCal days each week.

My energy levels have increased and I really appreciate my Indulgence days, making sure to include the occasional pastry, bar of chocolate and glass of wine without any of the guilt I once felt about such "treats" and knowing from experience that they do not interfere with my weight-loss program. As an extra bonus, I don't have to try to work out how to fit in the two recommended alcohol-free days each week. I know my glass of wine is high in calories so I don't include it in my LoCal days. This way I can appreciate it so much more when I do have a tipple!

I have considerably greater zest for life than before and look forward to each day of the healthier, happier, more productive life I'm leading. I wish you the same result!

As with any diet, it is important that if you have any ongoing health issues you should consult your doctor before proceeding.

Mindful Eating

I now want to look at just how we can make doing this diet really enjoyable by developing a truly mindful approach to it.

We spend a lot of time 'sleepwalking' through our lives; at least, I certainly do. What I mean by that is that, all too often, we are trying to multi-task or doing stuff on 'automatic pilot'.

How many times have you driven some place and wondered how you actually got there? That's not to suggest that you are a bad driver, it's just that things we do habitually like cleaning our teeth, dressing or everyday household chores frequently get done with our thoughts going off in different directions. Rarely are we completely focused on the task in hand.

Whilst getting showered in the morning I might be thinking about what I'm going to do later in the day, something I did yesterday or what to wear. That doesn't mean I don't wash properly! It does mean, though, that I am not completely aware of what I am doing.

There have also been too many times when I have visited the ladies' toilet (the rest room) in a restaurant and on exiting have mindlessly ended up in the staff kitchen or another toilet, simply because I didn't notice the route I came in by!

Thomas Edison, the inventor of the electric light bulb, once asked several of his long-term employees what they noticed every day walking along the path from the road to his factory. When they had finished telling him everything they had seen around them on that fine spring morning, he was astonished to find that not one of them had mentioned the beautiful flowering cherry tree to one side of the path.

We can get so used to *doing* things that we can actually miss out heavily on *experiencing* them.

If we are being mindful, we are paying attention to what is actually going on, we are fully aware and awake in this moment. And realistically that's all there is – the here and now.

By being present we begin to wake up to the sensation of really living instead of switching off and disappearing somewhere else with our minds. We aren't in the past or the future but *here*, where it's all happening!

That's all very well, you might be thinking, but I have so many things to get done and I can't possibly shut out all the thoughts filling my head up. But that's the point – don't even try to.

Pause right now to watch what is going on in your

mind whilst you are reading this page. Thoughts will come and go even in this short space of time but that's fine - just notice them passing through like clouds, refrain from making any judgement about them or getting caught up in their content and steer your focus gently back to this experience .

I suggest you read the next bit and then try it out for yourself, closing your eyes if it makes it easier for you. It's a very short exercise, lasting only a few minutes, which has helped me to be mindful and which will, I hope, be helpful to you.

First, be *aware* of and just observe what thoughts are in your mind - watch them; then explore and try to name what you are feeling emotionally (happy, worried, self-critical...) and whether you feel tension in any part of your body – jaw, shoulders, buttocks...

Now *redirect your focus* to your breath – following its journey from the moment it enters your nostrils, flows down your windpipe and expands your chest and abdomen, to its way out, noting any change in temperature as it exits your nose. If any thoughts crop up whilst you are doing this, just briefly acknowledge them rather than dwell on them and then return to your breath.

Finally, scan your entire body, including your posture and facial expression, and then *breathe into any muscular tension* allowing it to soften as you breathe out.

That's it! How do you feel now? Any different from before you began?

I try to practice this exercise about three times a day. It invariably ends up with my feeling more relaxed, more grounded in the present and at ease with myself. I also become conscious of how much I tend to tighten up physically, quite involuntarily, as well as my tendency to be hard on myself. For example, I have in the past told myself repeatedly that I was fat, putting myself down in a manner that would be extremely hurtful if I did it to others.

And remembering to be kind to yourself is important, perhaps especially so when you are trying to follow a diet.

Mindfulness is worth reading about in much greater detail as it is an important and extremely useful life skill. However, for the purpose of this book I have tried to explain it as simply as possible so that you grasp enough to apply it to your 5:2 diet.

There are a good number of 'Mindful Eating' courses in the UK, France and the USA which must mean there is a need to take a different view of the essential, habitual activity of food consumption.

I have certainly found that taking time to apply mindful practice to my meals has improved not merely my attitude to and appreciation of what I eat but has also enabled me to 'slow down' a little in other things I do, as opposed to tearing mindlessly through the day. Whenever I tackle any task mindfully I achieve so much more than if I rush through it with half an eye on whatever I have to do next.

So you could start your LoCal day with the breathing exercise and then set about preparing your first meal with awareness, being fully focused on what you are doing from the moment you select the ingredients for your meal, through preparing them with interest, to choosing the crockery and cutlery.

When everything is prepared, sit down at a table and eat *without* engaging in any other activities at the same time (reading the newspaper, watching TV, listening to the radio...).

Appreciate the juxtaposition and appearance of the combination of foods on your plate and the origin of the products. A different selection of colours can look really appealing and inviting. Thinking about the rain, sun and the farmers who helped produce what is in front of you can also make you thankful for it.

Notice each piece of food you select as you eat it: its colour, size, shape and smell. Pay attention to the texture and taste of it in your mouth and where on your tongue it tastes differently. And chew it slowly.

A meal concentrated on in this manner can be

surprisingly and pleasurably different from one that is hurried through or consumed whilst doing other things. Even a small amount can feel and taste good. And because you have slowed the process down it feels more filling and is excellent for your digestion.

When I approach my LoCal day like this it becomes infinitely more satisfying.

The Light of Experience

I have now been a devotee of the 5:2 diet for almost a year – far outstripping the length of time spent trying to follow a vast variety of other weight loss regimes over the years. My experience with every other diet had led me to believe that I simply did not have the necessary will power to stay permanently on any program. And each time I gave up I felt a sense of failure as my waistline expanded yet again. I became thoroughly fed up with my all-too-frequent pattern of yo-yo dieting.

As obesity runs in my natural family (I was adopted but managed to trace my birth mother – the subject of another book), I feared becoming morbidly obese, diabetic and dying prematurely as my mother sadly did.

Once I got to grips with the calories in different foods it became much easier to choose what to eat on my LoCal days. And the fact that I only have to calorie restrict for two days in a week has made it "do-able".

That is not to say, however, that it's been plain sailing all the time to date. And this is what I want to share with you in this section – the difficulties I've encountered and how I have dealt with them, then the small triumphs that have made it thoroughly worthwhile continuing.

Constipation and headaches were initially a problem which I quickly solved by drinking lots of water, fruit infusions and calorie-free green tea. Before I started the 5:2, green tea wasn't a beverage I would have rated but now I must confess to an addiction to it! Even on my 'Indulgence' days it's frequently my drink of choice. Hot drinks also helped greatly at times when, during winter, I felt particularly cold. Calories produce heat, so it's understandable that I might sometimes feel somewhat colder on LoCal days.

Spreading my 500 calories across the day, when my calorie intake is lower, means that I avoid the sudden energy dips that can occur as the body uses up its store of quick-release glucose.

Having my meals at regular intervals on a LoCal day and generally reserving a reasonable number of calories for my evening meal overcame the bouts of irritability and anxiety that I noticed creeping in when I tried skipping lunch or sometimes not bothering to have any food at all until evening.

Initially, I became pre-occupied with thoughts of food, especially when I felt a strong pang of hunger (this disappeared after a few weeks when I began to settle into the diet) or watched someone tucking into a tasty dessert. This is where a mindful approach helped tremendously. Not only did I remind myself that I too could have this the next day but I turned my mind to an activity which did not involve food, such as writing, reading or creating colourful pictures in my art studio (a posh name for a shed in the garden!).

In the beginning, I would wake up after a LoCal day and get myself a massive breakfast with the idea that, having eaten a lot less the previous day, I must need loads to fill me up. When I tried to get through the mound of cereal, toast and eggs I had prepared, I felt bloated and uncomfortable. I soon concluded that the amount of food I *thought* was necessary was utterly disproportionate to what I could *actually* manage. With time my stomach had begun to shrink and could not hold so much.

After a couple of months on the diet I was consistently finding that vegetables were an excellent way to fill me up on a low calorie day but that the amount of meat I was able to have seemed quite meagre. So I considered making my two days per week totally vegetarian. I set about exploring what sorts of foods were available. I soon discovered that not only was the range of options much greater than I had previously imagined (such as the vast choice of Quorn products) but that they tasted really good and their calorie content was almost always far lower than meat alternatives.

In fact, I now enjoy vegetarian meals to such an extent that I rarely stray from this healthy eating style on the other five days.

A particularly exciting find was almond milk, a beverage manufactured from ground almonds. It is an excellent substitute for dairy milk and massively lower in calories – especially the unsweetened variety. Using this frees up extra calories to add a bit more substance to a meal.

Being kind to myself if I am having a bad day, which might be completely unrelated to food, is an effective way to deal with any distress. In the past I often used food to comfort myself but then I discovered rather more healthy ways to make myself feel better. It might be a bit of retail therapy like treating myself to a dress to suit my size 14 figure (my UK size 16-18 clothes needed replacing). But more often it's something that costs nothing, like going into the garden or walking in the park, listening to the various sounds, feeling the sun warming my skin and looking at the beauty of nature around me. I don't try to push away any feelings inside me – I simply notice them and accept that they are there but am aware of the need to look outward as well.

Tiredness became a problem too, at times. So I stopped pushing myself to exercise on LoCal days and began taking space for some 'me' time – not easy when so many things need doing. I invariably find though, that I get far more done on a day where I am conscious of doing only one thing - such as eating - at any given moment and giving it my entire attention for the duration.

Like so many others on this diet, I am considerably slimmer, having now lost a total of 8 kilos (18 pounds). There have been a few fluctuations but I have now reached and am staying (within a whisker) at my target weight of 56 kilos (124 pounds). At one point I was concerned that my weight would continue to drop indefinitely but it has pretty much remained at a constant level for the past couple of months on this weight reducing (or nowadays, weight-maintenance) program.

I definitely have considerably more energy than I used to have and feel lighter and more contented. Whenever I see a photograph of myself taken a year or two ago, it reminds me of how much I have achieved with minimal effort.

As for cognitive improvement I can honestly say I feel more alert, though whether or not my memory has indeed improved could be debatable. I only know that it feels good!

The 5:2 diet is far from being a faddy one. In fact it's not so much a diet as a completely different view of what and how we eat. It's a whole new approach to food which I find extremely effective and satisfying (I even find myself looking forward to my LoCal days!). I finally feel in control of my eating patterns.

I am including my website address at the beginning of this book so that, if you wish, you can let me know how you are getting on. I would be very interested to hear your experiences and am happy to answer any questions you may have.

Menus for LoCal Days – Introduction

As I've already said, gourmet cooking is just not my "thing". It's not that I don't appreciate fine food, more that I don't really enjoy spending too much time in the kitchen. So in compiling the menus that follow, I tried to keep things simple. They were, after all, written initially for my own use and I've altered them very little for the purposes of this book.

As they stand, the menus are designed for a woman to follow. However, they are equally suitable for men, who have the advantage of being able to choose another 100 calories-worth of nutrition. If you are following the diet with a partner I would suggest that the man chooses something that isn't going to make the woman envious – or else eats his 100-calories-worth of chocolate or biscuits in private! Better still, settle on a selection of fruit. After all, there are still five other days in the week for treats...

Please note the use of the word "menus" in this section. With just a few exceptions, there are no recipes as such. I'm making the assumption that most of my readers know how to cook – probably better than I do! The question isn't "How?" but "What?". Therefore, I've given a good number of varied ideas to suit a wide variety of tastes. The "How?" of cooking I leave to you in the main!

It's important for any would-be dieter to be comfortable with the diet they follow, so I need to make the point here that nothing in these menus is "writ in stone". The whole idea of presenting the sample menus in this book is to give you a kick-start to the 5:2 diet without the effort of starting from scratch. Hopefully, it will also motivate you to continue. Eventually, familiarity with the calorific values will enable you to make informed choices for yourself. My own experience has been that after the first few weeks of planning, I began to build up a mental repertoire of calories based on what I was eating regularly.

If there are things in these menus that are not to your taste, the counter and chart at the end of the book will enable you to choose substitutes in a mix-and match fashion, bearing in mind the fact that this may well mean adjusting some of the other parts of a day's menu to take account of any changes in the calorific values for the day. To facilitate this, I've listed the calorific values for each ingredient, as well as for the meal as a whole.

This diet is an adjustment in lifestyle. For five days each week you don't have to count calories. Obviously you will want to eat a well-balanced diet, as we all should, but there's no point in denying yourself luxuries. On the two LoCal days, calorie counting is of course necessary but I want to stress here that it's important to understand that there is no need to get obsessed with numbers – the spirit of the diet is far more important than its minute details. Calorie-counting in the frenetic way I did on my third day of the 5:2 diet, would consume your mind as well as your time and is psychologically unhealthy. So if you are over or under by a few calories, there is no guilt attached. Commonsense should prevail and remind us that whoever came up with the numbers of calories to be consumed each day was not laying down some unbreakable law. Metabolic rates, the rate at which our bodies burn up energy, vary from person to person according to many factors, so there is nothing magic about the number 500 (or 600 for men). Certainly, from the viewpoint of getting the diet to work, we should aim to get reasonably close to these target numbers or we'll stray off course and little by little the whole purpose of the diet will be lost. But don't allow obsession to take over, either! In fact, as you'll notice, the daily totals of calories do not always amount to exactly 500.

At the end of the first page of menus ("Day 1") I've mentioned the need to drink water at regular intervals. This could have been added to every page but I didn't want to labour the point. It's enough to emphasise that drinking water is not only good for your system in many well-documented ways, but also really does help to alleviate hunger and keep at bay the headaches so often associated with lower food intake.

Like most British people I like my cup of tea. If you

share this taste, the fact that tea has zero calories means that you can indulge yourself even on LoCal days, though if you want milk in it you will have to factor it into your menu and allow for the extra calories. I've listed tea with milk in a couple of menus but to give you some idea of low or zero calorie alternatives I've included a wide variety of them. I wouldn't want you to get the idea that I'm recommending that you drink a different flavoured tea or infusion (sometimes called "fruit teas") for every meal – imagine the number of opened packets you'd have in your cupboard if you used all the teabags I've mentioned! If you find something you like, there's nothing wrong with sticking with it. I acknowledge here the fact that I raided the website of Twining's Tea to remind myself of some of these flavours.

That brings me to the issue of brand names. In writing this book I intended to steer clear of using brand names; having no connection or vested interests with any food company, I've no particular reason to favour one brand over another. However, occasionally I found it necessary to use such names to identify the type of product. Had I, for instance, mentioned "whole wheat biscuits" it might have caused confusion, whereas the word "Weetabix" is so well anchored in the public consciousness (at least in the UK) that its use clarifies the meaning instantly. But it should be borne in mind that alternative brands, including supermarkets' own, are equally acceptable and often cheaper. And, as you'll see from the sample menus, I added in just a couple of branded ready meals that I've tried for myself and enjoyed. Occasionally, if you're pressed for time, a low calorie ready meal is a viable option.

With vegetarian "meat substitute" products it is almost impossible not to name brands, since their formulation is often unique to one company or another. So to mention "vegetarian sausage" is not enough in itself as can be seen if you compare the calorific values of the Linda McCartney and Quorn varieties. This does not in any way imply, however, that any one brand is better than another, merely different.

The sweet-toothed among you will look in vain in these menus for chocolate or puddings; after all, the joy of the 5:2 diet is that these luxuries are permitted for the other five days in the week. However, there are those for whom having tea, coffee or cereal without a sweetener is a step too far. For them there is good news: there is a natural healthy sugar alternative, a sweetener that is produced from the leaves of the stevia plant (a member of the sunflower family), which is three times as sweet as sugar and is rated as having zero calories. It is readily available in supermarkets (in the UK it is under the brand name of Truvia).

When cooking, it's good to know that grilling, steaming or boiling add no calories to food. However, frying is a different matter: you have to take into account the amount of oil or fat used. Here again, a product has been developed for the calorie-conscious: a range of oil sprays can be found in most supermarkets, labelled "1-Cal". One spraying is equal to one calorie of oil. I use the olive oil spray but sunflower oil is also available. It should be borne in mind, of course, that you may need up to eight sprays to fry your food, but that's still only eight calories. And as one tablespoonful of regular olive oil weighs in at a hefty 120 calories, the benefit becomes immediately obvious.

As to weights and measures, I've tried to make it easy but even here it's necessary to bring in a note of caution: other than exact weights, a lot is open to interpretation. Sometimes a familiar term, meant to signify a measure, can be almost meaningless in reality. What exactly is a "pat" of butter? The question is not just a matter of being picky about words – since a "pat" is said to contain 35 calories, getting this wrong makes quite a substantial difference. After trawling the internet, I found that a "pat" is defined as being one inch square by a third of an inch thick. Perhaps there's an opening for someone who wants to go into business as a patmaker, making it easier to measure butter accurately!

And what exactly, for instance, constitutes a "medium" sized potato? On some websites this is given as a diameter – but potatoes also vary in length. A potato 2½ inches wide could be thought of as medium, as some websites suggest – but what if it's six feet long...?

I leave it to your good common sense to interpret words such as large, medium and small. Similarly, talking about measures such as teaspoons and tablespoons can seem quite arbitrary. So you can take it that within these pages a spoonful, whatever sized spoon it is, means a gentle heap, not a mini-mountain.

At this point I need to make the necessary disclaimer: whilst I have taken care to check all my figures relating to calorific values and to give information that is as accurate as possible, I do not guarantee that they are exact. Where manufacturers' figures are available, I have used them. Where my research has revealed a degree of disagreement on the calorific content of certain foods, I've steered a middle course, generally rounding up or down to the nearest five. For foodstuffs with a content of fewer than twenty calories I've aimed to be as accurate as possible.

One way to make your LoCal meals more interesting and appealing to the eye is to think about their presentation. To this end I have tried to vary the colours on your plate and a few sprigs of parsley, weighing in at a mere two calories or some mint leaves, which are virtually zero rated, not only add an extra bit of nourishment but also a lovely splash of colour as a garnish. Furthermore, current scientific research suggests that the various natural colours of foods indicate the type of nutrients they contain. So it would seem that the greater the range of colours we consume, the wider our intake of nutrients.

Treating each meal as a special event, presenting it artistically and eating it slowly, savouring each mouthful, will heighten your enjoyment and leave you feeling more satisfied. To remove the impression of a having too little on my plate I treated myself to a set of smallish but very attractive plates. A fairly full small plate has a far better psychological effect than a half-empty large one! And I reserve these plates for my LoCal days to make my meals feel special.

To make your life easier it will help if you have a few basic measuring implements to hand: such high-tech devices as a teaspoon, a tablespoon, a measuring jug and a set of scales capable of weighing grams or ounces.

Calorie Counter – Introduction

Sticking with a diet is made so much easier if you can find the information you need in one place. There may be some people who get a buzz from wandering round a supermarket and reading the information on the packaging but I'm sure there are far more who, like me, would prefer to have a basic reference guide to enable them to plan their meals quickly and simply.

To that end, I have devised a calorie counter, which you'll find on the last pages of this book, to help you to mix and match according to your taste, with a minimum of effort. It is not comprehensive: it's not meant to be. It is designed rather to give you a head start in making the 5:2 diet work for you. It lists only foods easily available in most supermarkets (I would have said *all* supermarkets but I don't want to tempt fate!).

Those with sharp eyes will notice that some foods appear in two lists: milk, for instance, is to be found under "Drinks" as well as under "Dairy" as it fits equally well into both.

As for the anomaly of soups in the Drinks list, I just didn't know where else to put them and the fact that many people like to drink their soup from a mug or cup suggested that this was the best place. And, yes, I know that tomatoes are, technically-speaking, a fruit but they usually get placed with vegetables in supermarkets so that's where I've put them in my counter!

What makes this counter particularly useful is that it is arranged in order of calorific values. That way, if you have planned your day's diet and find you are a few calories short of your 500 (or 600 if you're a man), you can refer to the relevant section to find a little more to top up on. For example, if you have a 20 calorie shortfall, looking in the section "11-20" will give you a choice of fruity treats or a bit of extra veg – or even a cup of tea with added milk. If you can't find anything in that section to meet your fancy, try looking at the section with double the calories: you may well find something there where halving the stated quantity will give you the number of calories you require.

The calorie content for each item is the number in brackets at the end of each line.

The calorie counter is followed by a chart listing foods in alphabetical order, giving the calorie content in a range of common weights and measures. It will prove a useful aid in getting to grips with "knowing your calories" and will give you an easy way to check on specific ingredients quickly. I've thrown in several extra items that you may find useful but which are not actually used in the menu pages. This gives you greater choice.

So now it's over to you. Enjoy! *Bon appétit!*

A brief note for American readers:

In the UK nowadays, metric measurements have become as commonplace as Imperial ones, possibly even more so. To make things a bit easier for you, it may help you to know that 28 grams are equal to one ounce (so 56 grams are 2 oz, 84 grams are 3 oz...) and that 1 fluid ounce equals 29.6 millilitres (ml) which is as close to 30ml as makes no difference (the remaining 0.4ml would be the drop that makes a tiny stain on your sweater!).

If a few of the brand names do not exist in the USA, I'm sure you will find plenty of suitable alternatives in your local supermarket. The calorie count is the important factor!

According to the writer George Bernard Shaw, the British and Americans are two nations *divided* by a common language. I am aware, for instance that the wispy green leaf we call "rocket", you call "arugula". Similarly, our "courgette" is your "zucchini", a name you borrowed from the Italians, whereas we copied the French. Whilst I've tried to keep this in mind and hope this book makes intelligent and intelligible sense to you, I hope also that you will be tolerant of any uniquely British words or expressions that may have crept in. They weren't intended to confuse you, really they weren't!

Sample Menus for 24 LoCal Days

Day 1

BREAKFAST
10g porridge oats (40 cal)
    60ml soya milk (30 cal)
    Stevia to sweeten (0 cal)
Microwave for 2 min (700W). Add blueberries 50g (25 cal)
Microwave for further 30 sec & serve. Timings are approximate and will vary according to the power of your microwave. For a smoother consistency add a little water as desired.

Green tea (0 cal)
Total calories 95

LUNCH
1 slice medium wholemeal bread, toasted (70 cal)
    Spread with 1 tsp peanut butter (30 cal)
1 small egg, boiled (55 cal)

Cup of tea with semi-skimmed milk (15 cal)
Total calories 170

DINNER
1 Quorn vegetarian burger, grilled (80 cal)
84g cauliflower (dry measure) steamed (50 cal)
1 medium carrot, steamed (25 cal)
84g peas, cooked from frozen (35 cal)
Garnish with 2 sprigs fresh parsley (1 cal)
Side salad:
    2 sticks celery (10 cal)
    6 cherry tomatoes (20 cal)
    6 slices cucumber (5 cal)
    112g lettuce (5 cal)

Apple Infusion (2 cal)
Total calories 233

TOTAL CALORIES FOR DAY: 498

Drink several glasses of water throughout the day

Day 2

BREAKFAST
Scrambled egg made with:
    1 large egg (75 cal)
    Semi-skimmed milk 10ml (5 cal)
    Half tsp butter (15 cal)
    Salt (0 cal)
    Black pepper (pinch) (0 cal)
1 crispbread (20 cal)
    Spread with ½ tsp peanut butter (15 cal)

Black tea with slice of lemon (1 cal)
Total calories 131

LUNCH
1 medium carrot (25 cal)
1 kiwi fruit (45 cal)
10 grapes (35 cal)

Glass of water (0 cal)
Total calories 105

DINNER
1 small (120g) potato, baked (110 cal)
    Top with 28g Cheddar cheese, grated (110 cal)
1 tsp onion, raw chopped (4 cal)
4 radishes (5 cal)
1 large red tomato, quartered (35 cal)

Green tea (0 cal)
Total calories 264

TOTAL CALORIES FOR DAY: 500

Day 3

BREAKFAST
1 medium slice wholemeal toast (75 cal)
>   *Top with* 112g canned chopped tomatoes, heated (25 cal)
>   *Garnished with* 5 fresh mint leaves (1 cal)

Green tea (0 cal)
Total calories 101

LUNCH
3 low-fat cream crackers (55 cal)
>   *Top with* 35g mini tub extra light Philadelphia cheese (38 cal)
84g grated carrot (25 cal)

Diet cola (0 cal)
Total calories 118

DINNER
Pasta Salad:
>   50g penne pasta   (dry weight) (175 cal)
>   35g peas, cooked from frozen (25 cal)
>   1 tsp chopped parsley (1 cal)
>   1 tsp chopped chives (1 cal)
>   Juice of ½ lemon (10 cal)
>   ½ tbsp olive oil (60 cal)
>   1 tbsp onion, chopped (10 cal)

Cook pasta & peas. Drain & rinse, combine & mix with other ingredients. Cover & store in fridge until required. Serve cold.

Sparkling water (0 cal)
Total calories 282

TOTAL CALORIES FOR DAY: 501

Day 4

BREAKFAST
10g porridge oats (40 cal)
    60ml soya milk (30 cal)
    Stevia to sweeten (0 cal)
Microwave for 2 min (based on 700W). Add 84g strawberries (25 cal)
Microwave for further 30 sec & serve. Timings are approximate and will vary according to the power of your microwave. For a smoother consistency add a little water as desired.

Lime & Ginger infusion (2 cal)
Total calories 97

LUNCH
1 large apple (110 cal)
1 kiwi fruit (45 cal)

Coffee, black filtered (2 cal)
Total calories 160

DINNER
56g falafel, cooked as per manufacturer's instructions (156 cal)
100g broccoli (35 cal)
100g sliced carrot (cooked or raw) (35 cal)
    Garnish with 3 sprigs parsley (1 cal)

Tea with semi-skimmed milk (15 cal)
Total calories 242

TOTAL CALORIES FOR DAY: 499

Day 5

BREAKFAST
1 medium egg, boiled (65 cal)
1 medium slice wholemeal toast (75 cal)
    Spread with 1 tsp peanut butter (30 cal)

Earl Grey tea (0 cal)
Total calories 170

LUNCH
Fresh fruit mixed salad:
    Small apple, 1 chopped (55 cal)
    Kiwi fruit, 1 peeled & sliced (45 cal)
    Strawberries, chopped, 84g (3 oz) (20 cal)
    Lemon juice 1 tsp (1 cal)

Diet cola (0 cal)
Total calories 121

DINNER
56g ready-marinated tofu pieces (127 cal)
112g prepacked stir-fry vegetables (60 cal)
    Stir-fry tofu and vegetables in 6 sprays of 1-cal olive oil (6 cal)
2 tbsp soy sauce (17 cal)

Green Tea (0 cal)
Total calories 210

TOTAL CALORIES FOR DAY: 501

Day 6

BREAKFAST
10g porridge oats (40 cal)
    60ml rice milk (30 cal)
Microwave for 2 min sec (700W). Add 84g of fresh raspberries (30 cal)
Microwave for further 30 sec & serve. Timings are approximate. For a smoother consistency add a little water as desired.

Black coffee, instant (2 cal)
Total calories 102

LUNCH
Hardboiled egg, large, sliced (75 cal)
Iceberg lettuce, 84g, shredded (10 cal)
2 low-fat (1%) crackers (35 cal)
    Spread with 1 triangle extra-light processed cheese (20 cal)
3 cherry tomatoes (10 cal)
Green tea (0 cal)
Total calories 150

DINNER
84g cauliflower, steamed (30 cal)
84g broccoli, steamed (33 cal)
100g new potatoes (uncooked weight), boiled (75 cal)
Ingredients for topping:
    112g quark (75 cal)
    2 tsp sour cream (15 cal)
    1 tbsp skimmed milk (10 cal)
    2 tsp chopped parsley (1)
    2 tsp chopped chives (1)
Mix topping ingredients thoroughly and pour over vegetables

Filtered black coffee (2 cal)
Total calories 245

TOTAL CALORIES FOR DAY: 498

Day 7

BREAKFAST
Weetabix, 1 biscuit (65 cal)
    75 ml almond milk, unsweetened (10 cal)
    Stevia extract to taste (0 cal)

Strawberry & mango infusion (2 cal)
Total calories 77

LUNCH
Leek & Potato cup soup, low fat, 1 sachet (55 cal)
3 cherry tomatoes (10 cal)
1 small peach (35 cal)

Sparkling water (0 cal)
Total calories 100

DINNER
1 Asda (Walmart) cheese & onion crispbake (289 cal)
cooked as per instructions on packaging
112g lettuce (5 cal)
84g beetroot, diced (25 cal)
28g sliced mushrooms (4 cal)

Green tea (0 cal)
Total calories 323

TOTAL CALORIES FOR DAY: 500

Day 8

BREAKFAST
28g corn flakes (110 cal)
> 75 ml almond milk, unsweetened (10 cal)
> Stevia to taste (0 cal)

Tea with skimmed milk (10 cal)
Total calories 130

LUNCH
Banana & Blueberry Smoothie:
> 240ml almond milk, unsweetened (32 cal)
> 56g blueberries (32 cal)
> ½ medium banana (52 cal)
> Stevia to sweeten if required (0 cal)

Mix all ingredients thoroughly in blender

Total calories 116

DINNER
112g Quorn Vegetarian Family Roast (118 cal)
112g (uncooked weight) dry roasted new potatoes (84 cal)
84g carrots, steamed (35 cal)
Asparagus, 4 spears, steamed (15 cal)
> *Garnish with* parsley, 3 sprigs (2 cal)

Green tea (0 cal)
Total calories 254

TOTAL CALORIES FOR DAY: 500

Day 9

BREAKFAST
1 medium slice wholemeal bread, toasted (75 cal)
1 medium egg, scrambled as Day 2 (86 cal)
Tomato, medium, halved & grilled (25 cal)

Coffee, black filtered (2 cal)
Total calories 188

LUNCH
3 stalks celery (15 cal)
Top with 70g cottage cheese, low fat (2%) (83 cal)
4 radishes (5 cal)

Black tea (0 cal)
Total calories 103

DINNER
50g (dry weight) spaghetti, cooked (156 cal)
½ of 390g carton chopped tomatoes, basil & oregano (53 cal)
Heat tomatoes and pour over spaghetti
Garnish with a teaspoon of chopped chives or sprig of parsley (1 cal)

Green tea (0 cal)
Total calories 210

TOTAL CALORIES FOR DAY: 501

Day 10

BREAKFAST
Banana smoothie:
>Yoghurt, plain, fat-free 150g pot (80 cal)
>Banana, small (70 cal)
>30ml almond milk, unsweetened (4 cal)
>½ tsp honey (10 cal)

Blend & serve

Green tea (0 cal)
Total calories 164

LUNCH
2 crispbreads (40 cal)
>*Spread with* 1 tsp Philadelphia light soft cheese (10 cal)
>*Top with* 6 slices cucumber (5 cal)

Sparkling water (0 cal)
Total calories 55

DINNER
Omelette:
>2 medium eggs (130 cal)
>1 small, diced onion (20 cal)
>½ yellow pepper, small, chopped (10 cal)
>Pinch of dried mixed herbs (1 cal)
>28g (1 oz) grated cheddar cheese (110 cal)
>2 tbsp water (0 cal)
>1 cal olive oil spray, 4 sprays (4 cal)

Serve with 112g leaf lettuce (6 cal)

Green tea & lemon (1 cal)
Total calories 282

TOTAL CALORIES FOR DAY: 501

Day 11

BREAKFAST
84g All-bran cereal (80 cal)
        75ml almond milk, unsweetened (10 cal)
        Stevia to taste (0 cal)

Black tea (0 cal)
Total calories 90

LUNCH
2 Ryvita slices original crispbread (40 cal)
        1 pat butter or margarine (35 cal)

Blueberry & Apple fruit infusion (2 cal)
Total calories 77

DINNER
Potato (about 200g), baked with skin (190 cal)
        Top with 112g low fat cottage cheese (110 cal)
        Garnish with teaspoon chopped chives (1 cal)
        2 small whole beet, cooked (30 cal)

Rooibos Red tea (0 cal)
Total calories 331

TOTAL CALORIES FOR DAY: 498

Day 12

BREAKFAST
½ grapefruit, sprinkled with stevia (40 cal)
1 medium slice white bread, toasted (55 cal)
    Low fat spread, 1 pat (35 cal)
    1 tsp marmalade (40 cal)

 Vanilla black tea (0 cal)
Total calories 170

LUNCH
10 grapes (35 cal)
2 small peaches (70 cal)
1 small apple (55 cal)
1 satsuma (20 cal)

Green tea with jasmine (0 cal)
Total calories 180

DINNER
Mixed salad:
Hardboiled egg, large sliced (75 cal)
    56g grated carrot (25 cal)
    84g diced beetroot (25 cal)
    ½ red pepper, small sliced (10 cal)
    ½ yellow pepper, small sliced (10 cal)
    84g iceberg lettuce, shredded (5 cal)

Black tea lemon spiced (0 cal)
Total calories 150

TOTAL CALORIES FOR DAY: 500

Day 13

BREAKFAST
10g porridge oats (40 cal)
        60ml semi skimmed milk (30 cal)
Microwave for 2 min sec (700W). Add 1 28g packet raisins (92 cal)
Microwave for further 30 sec & serve. Timings are approximate.
For a smoother consistency add a little water as desired.

English breakfast tea (black) (0 cal)
Total calories 162

LUNCH
2 rice cakes (60 cal)
        Spread with 1 tsp peanut butter (30 cal)

Ceylon Orange Pekoe tea (0 cal)
 Total calories 90

DINNER
1 Quorn vegetarian garlic & parsley sausage, grilled (104 cal)
        1 potato waffle, 56g (2 oz), grilled (95 cal)
        Small sliced onion, sautéed in 1 cal spray (24 cal)
        84g green beans, trimmed & cooked (25 cal)

Green tea with apple & pear (0 cal)
 Total calories 248

TOTAL CALORIES FOR DAY: 500

Day 14

BREAKFAST
Weetabix, 1 biscuit (65 cal)
    56g blackberries (24 cal)
    75ml almond milk, unsweetened (10 cal)
    Stevia to taste (0 cal)

Black tea (0 cal)
Total calories 99

LUNCH
1 slice medium wholemeal bread, toasted (75 cal)
1 pat butter or dairy-free spread (35 cal)
56g mushrooms fried in 5 sprays 1-cal oil (13 cal)
1 tomato, medium, grilled (25 cal)

Blackberry & Nettle Infusion (2 cal)
Total calories 150

DINNER
Salad:
10g watercress (2 cal)
2 sticks celery (10 cal)
6 cherry tomatoes (20 cal)
84g iceberg lettuce (5 cal)
3 spring onions (2 cal)
8 radishes (10 cal)
    Top with 1 tbsp cashew nuts, crushed (49 cal)
50g goat's cheese, sliced & grilled (150 cal)

Camomile, Fennel & Liquorice infusion (2 cal)
Total calories 250

TOTAL CALORIES FOR DAY: 499

Day 15

BREAKFAST
1 shredded wheat (75 cal)
    75ml almond milk, unsweetened (10 cal)
    Stevia to taste (0 cal)

Green tea (0 cal)
Total calories 87

LUNCH
2 slices Ryvita Original crispbread (40 cal)
    Topped with 28g low-fat cottage cheese (30 cal)

Lipton Morocco Mint & Spice infusion (3 cal)
Total calories 73

DINNER
1 Tesco nut cutlet (240)
    100g new potatoes, boiled (75 cal)
    56g peas, cooked from frozen (23 cal)
    Garnish with sprig of mint (0 cal)

Sparkling water (0 cal)
Total calories 338

TOTAL CALORIES FOR DAY: 498

Day 16

BREAKFAST
28g (1oz) Rice Krispies (110 cal)
    75ml semi-skimmed milk (37 cal)
    Stevia to taste

Aniseed, Fennel & Liquorice infusion (2 cal)
Total calories 149

LUNCH
1 medium banana (105 cal)
2 apricots (30 cal)
1 medium plum (30 cal)

Earl Grey tea (0 cal)
Total calories 165

DINNER
1 Linda McCartney Veg. Sausage (95 cal)
    ½ small red onion, sliced (10 cal)
Fry onion in 3 sprays 1-cal oil (3 cal)
    168g cabbage steamed (15 cal)
    84g new potatoes, boiled (63 cal)

Green tea (0 cal)
Total calories 186

TOTAL CALORIES FOR DAY: 500

Day 17

BREAKFAST
28g (1oz) cornflakes (110 cal)
    75ml skimmed milk (28 cal)
    Stevia if required (0 cal)

Green tea (0 cal)
Total calories 138

LUNCH
Strawberry, Lemon & Orange Smoothie:
    120ml fat-free vanilla yoghurt (64 cal)
    2 tsp lemon juice (1 cal)
    ¼ tsp lemon zest (0 cal)
    60ml orange juice (30 cal)
    112g strawberries (36 cal)
    Ice
    Blend all ingredients thoroughly

Total calories 131

DINNER
1 pack Quorn Cottage Pie, chilled ready meal, 300g (213 cal)
    6 slices cucumber (5 cal)
    3 cherry tomatoes (10 cal)
    2 sprigs parsley to garnish (1 cal)

Ginger infusion (2 cal)
Total calories 231

TOTAL CALORIES FOR DAY: 500

Day 18

BREAKFAST
28g (1oz) Grape nut cereal (100 cal)
    75ml almond milk, unsweetened (10 cal)

Black tea (0 cal)
Total calories 110

LUNCH
12 grapes (40 cal)
1 small peach (35 cal)
1 tangerine (35 cal)

Sparkling water (0 cal)
Total calories 110

DINNER
1 Quorn peppered steak (123 cal)
1 large tomato, grilled (35 cal)
1 small courgette (zucchini), sliced (15 cal)
1 small onion, sliced (20 cal)
116g new potatoes, sliced (87 cal)
Fry potatoes, courgette and onion gently in 8 sprays 1-cal oil (8 cal)

Green tea, lemon flavoured (0 cal)
Total calories 280

TOTAL CALORIES FOR DAY: 500

Day 19

BREAKFAST
1 crumpet, toasted (90 cal)
Spread with 1 tsp honey (20 cal)

Blackcurrant, Ginseng & Vanilla infusion (2 cal)
Total calories 112

LUNCH
3 sticks celery (15 cal)
With dip of:
1 mini tub extra light Philadelphia soft cheese, 35g (38 cal)
1 medium orange (60 cal)
1 medium pear (50 cal)

Sparkling water (0 cal)
Total calories 163

DINNER
56g feta cheese (148 cal)
6 cherry tomatoes (20 cal)
12 slices cucumber, (10 cal)
4 radishes (5 cal)
5 basil leaves, torn (1 cal)
A few flat parsley leaves (1 cal)
28g rocket (*arugula* in USA) (5 cal)
½ small red onion, sliced (10 cal)
¼ yellow pepper, sliced (5 cal)
Drizzle with:
1 tsp olive oil (20 cal)
1 tsp lemon juice (0 cal)

Green tea (0 cal)
Total calories 225

TOTAL CALORIES FOR DAY: 500

Day 20

BREAKFAST
1 large boiled egg (75 cal)
1 slice crispbread, (20 cal)
    S*pread with* 1 tsp peanut butter (30 cal)

Strawberry & mango infusion (2 cal)
Total calories 127

LUNCH
Cup-a Soup, spring vegetable, 13g sachet (45 cal)
3 sticks celery (15 cal)

Coffee, black filtered (2 cal)
Total calories 62

DINNER
2 Tivall vegetarian frankfurters (140 cal)
    84g peas (35 cal)
    112g potato, mashed with skimmed milk (130 cal)
    Mustard 1 tsp (5 cal)
    Garnish with 2 sprigs parsley (1 calorie)

Black tea (0 cal)
Total calories 311

TOTAL CALORIES FOR DAY: 500

Day 21

BREAKFAST
1 small egg (55 cal)
    Fry in 1-cal olive oil spray, 2 sprays (2 cal)
1 slice wholemeal bread, toasted (70 cal)
    S*pread with* 1 tsp olive spread (25 cal)

Black tea (0 cal)
Total calories 152

LUNCH
168g strawberries (45 cal)
    Top with 1 tbsp quark (15 cal)
    Mix with 2 drops vanilla essence (1 cal)
Stevia to taste (0 cal)

Blueberry & Apple infusion (2 cal)
Total calories 63

DINNER
100g Taifun smoked tofu, sliced (185 cal)
1 tsp crushed garlic (5 cal)
    Fry garlic and tofu together briefly in 4 sprays 1-cal oil (4 cal)
    Sprinkle with 2 tsp teriyaki sauce (10 cal)
200g broccoli, steamed (80 cal)

Green tea with slice of lemon (1 cal)
Total calories 285

TOTAL CALORIES FOR DAY: 500

Day 22

BREAKFAST
10g porridge oats (40 cal)
    Soya milk 60ml (30 cal)
    Stevia extract to sweeten (0 cal)
Microwave for 1 min 30 sec. Add 84g raspberries (30 cal)
Microwave for further 30 sec & serve. Timings are approximate.
For a smoother consistency add a little water.

Earl Grey tea (0 cal)
Total calories 100

LUNCH
2 rice cakes (60 cal)
    Top with 1 triangle extra light processed cheese, (20 cal)
6 slices cucumber (5 cal)

Sparkling water (0 cal)
Total calories 85

DINNER
"Easy Bean" Moroccan Tagine ready meal (211 cal)
    75g cooked long-grain rice (100 cal)
    112g iceberg lettuce (5 cal)

Diet cola (0 cal)
Total calories 316

TOTAL CALORIES FOR DAY: 501

Day 23

BREAKFAST
1 medium slice white bread, toasted (55 cal)
112g Heinz baked beans (reduced salt & sugar) (78 cal)

Green tea (0 cal)
Total calories 133 cal

LUNCH
1 small peach (35 cal)
12 cherries (60 cal)
1 medium plum (30 cal)
1 apricot (15 cal)

Diet cola (0 cal)
Total calories 140

DINNER
150g fresh egg noodles (102 cal)
150g prepacked oriental stir-fry vegetables (86 cal)
1 tbsp sweet chilli sauce (30 cal)
Fry noodles and vegetables in 8 sprays 1-cal oil (8 cal)
Splash with sauce immediately before removing from pan

Sparkling water (0 cal)
Total calories 226

TOTAL CALORIES FOR DAY: 499

Day 24

BREAKFAST

1 slice medium white bread, toasted (55 cal)
    Top with 112g chopped tomatoes, heated (25 cal)
    Garnish with 2 sprigs parsley (1 cal)

Options low fat chocolate drink (40 cal)
Total calories 120

LUNCH

1 medium Asian pear, fresh (50 cal)
1 small apple (55 cal)
100g honeydew melon (30 cal)
1 small peach (35 cal)

Sparkling water (0 cal)
Total calories 170

DINNER

Sweet Pepper,Tomato & Onion Omelette:
    2 small eggs (110 cal)
    1 tsp diced onion (4 cal)
    ½, yellow pepper, chopped (10 cal)
    ½ red pepper, chopped (10 cal)
    ½ green pepper, chopped (10 cal)
    6 cherry tomatoes, halved (20 cal)
    1 tsp olive/vegetable oil (40 cal)
    Salt & pepper (0 cal)
    Parsley garnish, 3 sprigs (1 cal)
Sauté peppers, tomatoes & onions lightly in oil, then pour on beaten eggs. Cook, garnish & serve

Camomile & Spear mint infusion (2 cal)
Total calories 207

TOTAL CALORIES FOR DAY: 497

Calorie Counter

0 – 10 Calories

Vegetables

Mint leaves (**0**)
Chives, 1 tsp chopped (**1**)
Mixed herbs, dried, 1 pinch (**1**)
Onion, 1 tsp raw chopped (**4**)
Mushrooms, 28g (1 oz) (**4**)
Parsley, 10 sprigs (**5**)
Cucumber, 6 slices (**5**)
Celery, 1 stick (**5**)
Garlic, 1 clove (**5**)
Radishes, 4 (**5**)
Iceberg lettuce, 112g (**5**)
Spring onions, 6 (**5**)
Leaf lettuce 112g (**5**)

Dairy

Sour cream, 1 tsp (**8**)

Drinks

Black tea (**0**)
Earl Grey tea (**0**)
Green tea (**0**)
Diet cola (**0**)
Twinings infusions (**2**)
Coffee, black (**2**)
Tea w/skimmed milk (**10**)

Miscellaneous

Salt (**0**)
Vinegar (**0**)
Stevia extract (sweetener) (**0**)
Mustard 1 tsp (**5**)
Soy Sauce 1 tbsp (**9**)

11 – 20 Calories

Vegetables

Cabbage, 112g (**15**)
Asparagus, 4 spears (**15**)
Courgette (zucchini),, 1 small (**15**)
Onion, 1 small (**20**)
Cherry tomatoes, 6 (**20**)
Sweet Pepper, 1 any colour (**20**)

Fruit

Plum, 1 medium (**30**)
Lemon, 1 medium (**15**)
Apricot 1 (**15**)
Satsuma 1 (**20**)

Dairy

Quark, 1oz (**19**)
Cheese triangle, extra light (**20**)

Drinks

Almond milk, unsweetened, 100ml (**10**)
Tea w/ semi-skimmed milk (**15**)
Tea w/ whole milk (**20**)

Miscellaneous

Ketchup, 1 tbsp (**15**)
Honey, 1 tsp (**20**)
Ryvita Original, 1 crispbread (**20**)

21 – 30

Vegetables

Tomato, 1 medium **(25)**
Carrot, 1 medium **(25)**
Beet, 2 small whole cooked **(30)**
Cauliflower, dry, 84g **(30)**

Fruit

Blueberries, 50g **(25)**
Melon, Honeydew 100g **(30)**

Dairy

Olive spread, 1 tsp **(25)**
Cottage cheese, low fat 28g **(30)**

Miscellaneous

Sugar, white, 1 tsp **(25)**
Rice cake, 1 **(30)**
Peanut butter, 1 tsp **(30)**
Sweet chilli sauce, 1 tbsp **(30)**

31 – 40

Vegetables

Onion, sliced, 168g (**40**)
Trimmed cut green beans, 168g (**40**)

Fruit

Pineapple, canned in juice, 1 ring (**35**)
Grapes, 10 (**35**)
Plum, 1 large (**35**)
Peach, 1 small fresh (**35**)
Tangerine, 1 small (**35**)
Grapefruit, half (**40**)
Apricots, canned in juice, 3 halves (**40**)

Dairy

Butter / margarine, 1 pat (**35**)
Extra Light Philadelphia soft cheese, 35g mini tub (**38**)

Drinks
Soya milk light, 120ml (**35**)
Options low fat chocolate drink, 1 serving (**40**)
Tomato juice, 120ml (**40**)

Miscellaneous

Cream crackers, low fat, 2 (**35**)
Marmalade / Jam, 1 tsp (**40**)

41 - 50

Vegetables

Broccoli, 112g (**45**)
Carrots, grated 112g (**45**)
Beet, cooked & diced, 168g (**50**)
Tomatoes, canned, chopped, 168g (**50**)

Fruit

Watermelon cubed, 168g (**45**)
Kiwi Fruit, 1 (**45**)
Strawberries, 168g (**45**)
Cherries, 10 (**50**)
Pear, Asian, 1 medium (**50**)

Drinks

Spring vegetable cup soup, 13g sachet (**45**)

51 – 100

Meat Alternatives

Frankfurter, vegetarian (Tivall), 1 (**70**)
Quorn vegetarian burger, 1 (**80**)
Linda McCartney vegetarian sausage, 1 (**95**)
Quorn vegetarian family roast, 112g (**118**)
Falafel, 56g, 1 (**156**)

Vegetables

Stir-fry vegetables, prepacked, 112g (60 cal)
Peas, cooked from frozen, 168g (**65**)
Carrots, cooked, 168g (**70**)
New potatoes, boiled, 100g (**75**)
Stir-fry vegetables, oriental prepacked, 150g (**86 cal**)
Potato waffle, 1 (56g) (**95**)
Corn on the cob, 1 medium (**100**)

Fruit

Apple, 1 small (**55**)
Orange, 1 medium (**60**)
Apples, peeled & sliced, 168g (**65**)
Raspberries, 168g (**65**)
Banana, small (**70**)
Sunmaid raisins, 1 small packet (28g) (**92**)

Dairy

Egg, 1 small (**55**)
Egg, 1 medium (**65**)
Egg, 1 large (**75**)
Yoghurt, fat-free plain, 150g pot (**80**)
Goat's cheese, 28g (**84**)
Milk, skimmed, 240ml (**77**)
Egg, 1 large, scrambled or omelette (**100**)

Cereals

Weetabix, 1 biscuit **(65)**
All-Bran cereal, 84g **(80)**
Grape Nuts cereal, 28g **(100)**
Shredded Wheat, 28g **(100)**

Drinks

Leek & Potato cup soup, low fat, 1 sachet **(55)**
Soya milk, 100ml **(55)**
Ovaltine light, 20g serving **(72)**
Red wine, 100ml **(75)**
White wine, 100ml **(80)**
Milk, skimmed, 240ml **(77)**
Grapefruit juice, 240ml **(95)**
Orange juice, 120ml **(100)**

Miscellaneous

Lemon juice, 240ml**(60)**
Honey, 1 tbsp **(65)**
Wholemeal bread, 1 medium slice **(75)**
Crumpet, 1 **(90)**
Peanut butter 1 tbsp **(95)**
Almonds, 14 **(100)**
Rice, white long-grain, 75g (cooked weight) **(100)**

101 – 200

Meat Alternatives

Quorn garlic & parsley sausage, 1 (**104**)
Quorn vegetarian British sausage, 1 (**111**)
Quorn peppered steak (**123**)
Tofu pieces ready-marinated 56g (**127**)
Tofu, smoked (Taifun), 100g (**185**)

Vegetables

Parsnips, cooked, 168g (**125**)
Potato, baked w/skin, 200g (**190**)
Baked beans, half can (**195**)
Potato, mashed w/skimmed milk, 168g (**200**)

Fruit

Banana, 1 medium (**105**)
Apple, 1 large (**110**)
Dried prunes, 5 large (**115**)

Dairy

Cheddar cheese, grated, 28g (**110**)
Milk, semi-skimmed, 240ml (**120**)
Yoghurt, low fat, flavoured, 125g pot (**125**)
Milk, whole, 240ml (**150**)

Cereals

Rice Crispies, 28g (**110**)
Corn flakes, 28g (**110**)
Muesli original, 45g (**170**)

Drinks

Milk, semi-skimmed, 240ml **(120)**
Milk, whole, 240ml **(150)**
Chicken soup, cream of, canned, 240ml **(190)**

Miscellaneous

Egg noodles, fresh, 150g **(102 cal)**
Macaroni, cooked, 168g (from 84g dry) **(115)**
Olive oil/vegetable oils, 1tbsp **(125)**
Muffin, 1 **(140)**
Peanuts, oil roasted, 28g **(150)**
Cashew nuts, dry roasted, 28g **(165)**
Penne pasta, 50g (dry weight) **(175)**
Brazil nuts, 28g **(185)**
Brown rice, long grain, 50g (dry weight) **(185)**
Bagel, 1 **(200)**

Over 200

Meat Alternatives

Moroccan Tagine ready meal (Easy Bean) **(211 cal)**
Quorn Cottage Pie, ready-meal 300g **(213)**
Nut cutlet, Tesco **(240)**
Cheese & onion crispbake, 1 - Asda (Walmart) **(289 cal)**

Calorie Chart: Alphabetical Order

Ingredient	1 item	28g (1 oz)	30ml (1 fl.oz)	1 Teaspoon	1 Tablespoon
All-Bran cereal		27			
Almond extract				11	
Almond milk, unsweetened			3		
Almonds, 14	100				
Apple, large	110				
Apple, medium	80	15			
Apple, small	55				
Apple juice			15		
Apricots, canned		14			
Apricot, fresh	15				
Asparagus spear	4				
Avocado	322	50			
Bagel	200				
Baked beans		20			
Banana, medium	105	25			
Banana, small	70	25			
Beans, green trimmed, cut		7			
Beet leaves	7	8			
Beetroot, cooked		12			
Beetroot, raw		12			
Berries, mixed		14			
Blackberries		12			
Blueberries		14			
Brazil nuts		185			
Bread, wholemeal, medium, per slice	75				

Ingredient	1 item	28g (1 oz)	30ml (1 fl.oz)	1 Teaspoon	1 Tablespoon
Broccoli		9			
Butter / margarine, 1 pat	35				
Cabbage		4			
Carrot	25	12			
Carrot juice			12		
Cashew nuts, dry roasted		165			
Cauliflower, dry		10			
Cayenne pepper				6	
Celery stalk	5	4			
Cheese, Cheddar, grated,		110			
Cheese triangle, extra light	20				
Cherries, frozen, de-stoned		13			
Cherry	5				
Chilli sauce, sweet					30
Chives, chopped				1	
Choc drink, Options low fat, serving	40				
Cinnamon, ground				6	
Cloves, ground				6	
Cocoa powder, unsweetened				4	12
Coconut water			6		
Coffee, brewed, black			1		
Coffee, instant granules, black				2	
Cola, diet			0		
Corn flakes		110			
Corn on the cob, medium	100				

Ingredient	1 item	28g (1 oz)	30ml (1 fl.oz)	1 Teaspoon	1 Tablespoon
Cottage cheese, low fat 28g		30			
Courgette (zucchini), small	15				
Cranberries		13			
Cranberry juice			15		
Cream crackers, low fat, 2	35				
Crumpet	90				
Cucumber, peeled	24	3			
Egg, large	75				
Egg, medium	65				
Egg, small	55				
Egg noodles, fresh		19			
Falafel		78			
Feta Cheese		74			
Frankfurter, vegetarian (Tivall)	70				
Fruit infusions (fruit teas), serving	2				
Garlic, 1 clove	5				
Ginger, ground				6	18
Ginger, root		22		2	
Goat's cheese		84			
Granola		95			35
Grape Nuts cereal		100			
Grapefruit	72				
Grapefruit juice			12		
Grapes		20			

Ingredient	1 item	28g (1 oz)	30ml (1 fl.oz)	1 Teaspoon	1 Tablespoon
Honey				20	60
Ice		0			
Kale leaves		14			
Ketchup					15
Kiwi fruit	29	13			
Leek & Potato cup soup, low fat, sachet	55				
Lemon without peel	17				
Lemon juice			7		4
Lemon zest				1	
Lettuce, iceberg		1			
Lettuce, leaf		1			
Lime juice			8	1	4
Macaroni, cooked		49			
Mango juice			15		
Marmalade / Jam				40	
Mango pieces, frozen		17			
Melon, cantaloupe		10			
Melon, honeydew		10			
Milk, skimmed			10		
Mint, fresh					1
Mixed herbs, dried, 1 pinch	1				
Muesli, Alpen original		109			
Muffin	140				
Mushrooms		4			
Mustard				5	

Ingredient	1 item	28g (1 oz)	30ml (1 fl.oz)	1 Teaspoon	1 Tablespoon
Nectarine	60				
Nut cutlet, Tesco	240				
Nutmeg, ground				12	36
Oatmeal					18
Oats, porridge		112			
Olive spread				25	
Olive oil / vegetable oils				40	120
Onion, chopped		7		1	4
Onion, small	20				
Orange	62				
Orange, large	86				
Orange juice			15		
Ovaltine light, serving	72				
Papaya, small	59	11			
Parsley		10			1
Parsnips, cooked		21			
Passion fruit	17				
Pasta, (dry weight)		98			
Peach nectar			17		
Peach, fresh	35				
Peanut butter, smooth				30	90
Peanuts, oil roasted		150			
Pear	96				
Pear, small	80				
Pear, Asian, medium	50				

Ingredient	1 item	28g (1 oz)	30ml (1 fl.oz)	1 Teaspoon	1 Tablespoon
Peas, cooked from frozen		12			
Pepper, ground				5	
Pepper, sweet (bell), any colour	20				
Philadelphia Extra Light, 35g mini tub	38				
Pineapple juice			17		
Pineapple, canned		17			
Pineapple, fresh		14			
Plum, medium	30				
Plum, 1 large	35				
Pomegranate juice			17		
Potato, baked w/skin, 200g	190				
Potato, mashed w/skimmed milk		33			
Potatoes new, boiled		21			
Prune juice			22		
Prunes, dried, large	23				
Quark		19			15
Quorn Garlic & Parsley Sausage	104				
Quorn Cottage Pie, ready meal, 300g	213				
Quorn Peppered Steak	123				
Quorn Veg British Sausage	111				
Quorn Veg Family Roast		30			
Radishes, 4	5				
Raisins, Sunmaid, pkt (28g)	92				

Ingredient	1 item	28g (1 oz)	30ml (1 fl.oz)	1 Teaspoon	1 Tablespoon
Raspberries		15			
Rhubarb pieces		6			
Rhubarb stalk	11				
Rice cake	30				
Rice milk			15		
Rice, brown long grain, (dry weight)		104			
Rice, white long-grain (cooked weight)		37			
Rice cake	30				
Rice Crispies		110			
Rocket (arugula)		4			
Salt		0		0	
Satsuma	20				
Sausage, Linda McCartney Vegetarian	95				
Shredded Wheat, 1 biscuit	75				
Sorbet, orange		25			
Sour cream				8	24
Soy sauce					9
Soya milk, sweetened			16		
Soya milk, unsweetened			8		
Soya milk, vanilla			14		
Spinach		7			
Spring onions, 6	5				
Spring veg cup soup sachet	45				
Strawberries		9			

Ingredient	1 item	28g (1 oz)	30ml (1 fl.oz)	1 Teaspoon	1 Tablespoon
Stevia		0		0	0
Sugar, white				25	
Tabasco sauce				1	
Tangerine	35				
Tea, green, serving	0				
Tea, Earl Grey, serving	0				
Tea, black, serving	0				
Tea w/skimmed milk, serving	10				
Tea w/ whole milk, serving	20				
Tea w/ semi-skimmed milk	15				
Tofu, ready-marinated		64			
Tofu, smoked (Taifun)		52			
Tomato, medium	25	5			
Tomatoes, cherry, 6	20	5			
Tomato, small	18	5			
Tomato juice			10		
Tomatoes, canned, chopped		8			
Vanilla essence				2	
Vanilla extract				12	
Vinegar				0	0
Waffle, potato, 56g	95				
Walnuts		194			40
Water		0		0	0
Watercress		4			
Watermelon		9			

Ingredient	1 item	28g (1 oz)	30ml (1 fl.oz)	1 Teaspoon	1 Tablespoon
Weetabix, biscuit	65				
Yeast extract (Marmite)				10	
Yoghurt, lemon, fat-free		24			12
Yoghurt, natural, fat-free		16			8
Yoghurt, vanilla, fat-free		16			8

4646299R00053

Printed in Great Britain
by Amazon.co.uk, Ltd.,
Marston Gate.